RISING TO THE OCCASION

," A GROUNDBREAKING BOOK THAT DELVES INTO THE SENSITIVE YET PREVALENT ISSUE OF ERECTILE DYSFUNCTION

ALEX USIFO

*To every individual and couple facing the challenges of erectile
dysfunction,
May this book serve as a guiding light on your journey to
understanding, acceptance, and triumph. Your courage in
confronting this common yet often stigmatized issue is inspiring.
This work is dedicated to those who dare to seek solutions,
embrace vulnerability, and strive for a renewed sense of intimacy.
In the face of adversity, may you find strength; in moments
of doubt, may you discover resilience; and in the pursuit of
connection, may you uncover a path towards a fulfilling and
empowered life.
This book is for you, with the sincere hope that it brings comfort,
knowledge, and a renewed sense of possibility.
With empathy and encouragement*

CONTENTS

INTRODUCTION

In a world where relationships thrive on emotional connection and physical intimacy, erectile dysfunction (ED) can pose a significant challenge. It affects millions of men worldwide and can take a toll not only on their physical well-being but also on their self-esteem and relationships. If you're grappling with ED or seeking knowledge to help a loved one, you've taken the first step toward finding a solution.

"Healing Intimacy" is your guide to understanding, addressing, and ultimately conquering erectile dysfunction through a holistic approach. This book combines the best of both worlds: the wisdom of traditional herbal remedies and the advancements of modern medical science to provide you with a comprehensive toolkit for restoring your sexual vitality.

Erectile dysfunction is a multifaceted issue that can be caused by various factors, including physical, psychological, and emotional elements. While prescription medications like Viagra have become popular solutions, they may not be suitable for everyone. Herbal remedies, lifestyle changes, and alternative therapies offer additional avenues for those looking to regain control of their sexual health.

Throughout the pages of "Healing Intimacy," we will explore the causes of ED, the medical treatments available, and the science behind herbal remedies. You'll learn about lifestyle modifications, dietary changes, and the importance of emotional well-being in your journey to overcoming ED. By blending the wisdom of herbal medicine with the expertise of medical science, you can develop a personalized plan to address your unique needs.

This book also delves into the importance of open communication with your partner and provides guidance on how to navigate this intimate challenge together. After all, relationships thrive on trust, empathy, and the ability to face life's challenges as a team.

Whether you're experiencing ED firsthand or seeking to support a loved one, "Healing Intimacy" offers a wealth of information, practical advice, and case studies to help you make informed decisions. By addressing this issue head-on, you can rediscover the joy and satisfaction that physical intimacy can bring to your life.

Remember, you're not alone on this journey. With the right knowledge, determination, and support, you can reclaim your sexual vitality and strengthen the bonds of intimacy that make life rich and fulfilling. Let's embark on this journey together, as we explore the path to healing intimacy and overcoming erectile dysfunction.

MEDICAL APPROACHES TO ERECTILE DYSFUNCTION

Erectile dysfunction (ED) is a common issue that affects men of various ages and backgrounds. It can be caused by a range of factors, both physical and psychological. While many people explore herbal and lifestyle remedies, it's important to be aware of the medical approaches available to address ED. In this chapter, we'll delve into the conventional medical treatments, prescription medications, hormone therapy, and other interventions that can help you regain control of your sexual health.

1. Conventional Medical Treatments

Conventional medical treatments for ED often involve procedures that directly address the physiological causes of erectile dysfunction. These treatments are typically recommended by healthcare professionals and may include:

Penile Pumps: A vacuum erection device, also known as a penile pump, is a non-invasive option. It involves placing a tube over the penis and using a pump to create a vacuum, which draws blood into the penis and produces an erection.

Penile Implants: For more severe cases of ED, a penile implant may be recommended. This surgical procedure involves placing inflatable or malleable rods into the penis, allowing for controlled erections.

2. Prescription Medications

The introduction of prescription medications revolutionized the treatment of erectile dysfunction. Here are some of the most commonly prescribed drugs for ED:

Sildenafil (Viagra): Sildenafil is one of the most well-known and widely used medications for ED. It works by increasing blood flow to the penis, helping achieve and maintain an erection. It's taken as needed, usually about 30 minutes before sexual activity.

Tadalafil (Cialis): Tadalafil is another popular medication for ED. It has a longer duration of action compared to sildenafil, allowing for more spontaneity in sexual activity. It can be taken daily or as needed.

Vardenafil (Levitra) and Avanafil (Stendra): These are other PDE5 inhibitors similar to sildenafil and tadalafil, offering options for individuals who may not respond well to one medication.

3. Hormone Therapy

Hormone imbalances, particularly low testosterone levels, can contribute to erectile dysfunction. Hormone therapy, which may include testosterone replacement, can help address this underlying issue and improve sexual function.

4. Counseling and Therapy

Psychological factors often play a significant role in ED. Individual or couples' counseling can be an essential part of treatment, especially when the root cause is anxiety, stress, or relationship issues. Therapy helps individuals and couples address emotional and psychological barriers to intimacy.

5. Surgical Options

In some cases, ED may be linked to structural issues. Surgical interventions, such as vascular surgery to improve blood flow, can be considered as a treatment option when other methods have been unsuccessful.

Medical approaches to ED offer a wide range of options to suit different needs and circumstances. It's crucial to consult with a healthcare professional to determine the most appropriate treatment plan. As you explore these options, remember that ED is a common and treatable condition, and there is hope for improvement in your sexual health. In the following chapters, we will further explore herbal remedies, lifestyle changes, and the importance of open communication with your partner as part of a

holistic approach to overcoming ED.

HERBAL REMEDIES FOR ERECTILE DYSFUNCTION

Herbal remedies have been used for centuries to address a variety of health concerns, including erectile dysfunction (ED). While herbal treatments are not a quick fix and may not work for everyone, many individuals find relief and improvements in their sexual health through natural approaches. In this chapter, we'll explore some of the most well-known herbal remedies for ED and their potential benefits.

1. Ginseng

Ginseng has been used in traditional medicine for its potential to improve sexual function and vitality. It is believed to work by promoting the release of nitric oxide, which relaxes and dilates blood vessels in the penis, allowing for increased blood flow and better erections.

2. L-Arginine

L-arginine is an amino acid that plays a role in the production of nitric oxide. Some studies suggest that L-arginine supplements may help improve blood flow to the penis, leading to better erections. It can be found in foods like nuts, seeds, and dairy products.

3. Ginkgo Biloba

Ginkgo biloba is an herbal remedy known for its potential to enhance blood circulation, which can be beneficial for individuals with ED. It may improve blood flow to the penis, leading to improved sexual function.

4. Maca Root

Maca root is a plant native to the Andes, and its root has been used for its potential aphrodisiac effects. It is believed to balance hormones, reduce stress, and increase energy levels, all of which can contribute to better sexual function.

5. Other Herbal Remedies

In addition to the above, there are several other herbal remedies that have been explored for their potential benefits in managing ED:

Yohimbe

Horny Goat Weed

Tribulus Terrestris

Saw Palmetto

Muira Puama

Tongkat Ali

It's important to note that while herbal remedies may offer

potential benefits, they can also come with side effects or interactions with other medications. If you're considering herbal remedies for ED, it's essential to consult with a healthcare professional to ensure they are safe and suitable for your individual circumstances.

Herbal remedies are just one part of the holistic approach to addressing erectile dysfunction. In the following chapters, we'll explore lifestyle and dietary changes that can support your journey to improved sexual health, as well as the importance of open communication with your partner and healthcare provider as you explore these natural alternatives.

LIFESTYLE AND DIET FOR
SEXUAL WELLNESS

Achieving and maintaining sexual wellness goes beyond just medical and herbal interventions. Your lifestyle and dietary choices play a significant role in supporting your sexual health. In this chapter, we'll explore the importance of nutrition, exercise, managing stress, quality sleep, and other lifestyle factors that can contribute to your overall well-being and sexual vitality.

1. Nutrition and Dietary Choices

A balanced and nutritious diet can positively impact your sexual health. Here are some dietary considerations:

- Fruits and Vegetables: Incorporate a variety of fruits and vegetables into your diet, as they are rich in antioxidants, vitamins, and minerals that promote overall well-being.

- Lean Proteins: Opt for lean protein sources like poultry,

fish, and legumes, as they can support muscle health and energy levels.

- Whole Grains: Choose whole grains such as brown rice, whole wheat, and oats to provide sustained energy and fiber.

- Healthy Fats: Include sources of healthy fats like avocados, nuts, and olive oil, which are important for hormone production.

- Hydration: Staying well-hydrated is crucial for overall health, including sexual function.

2. Exercise and Physical Activity

Regular physical activity has numerous benefits for sexual wellness:

- Cardiovascular Health: Exercise supports a healthy heart and blood circulation, which are essential for achieving and maintaining erections.

- Weight Management: Maintaining a healthy weight can help reduce the risk of ED, as excess weight can contribute to hormonal imbalances and reduced blood flow.

- Stress Reduction: Exercise is an effective way to reduce stress and anxiety, which can negatively impact sexual function.

3. Managing Stress and Mental Health

Stress and anxiety can be significant contributors to erectile dysfunction. Strategies to manage stress and support mental health include:

- Mindfulness and Meditation: These practices can help you stay present and reduce the impact of stressors.
- Therapy and Counseling: Seeking professional help to address emotional and psychological challenges can be beneficial.

4. Quality Sleep

- Getting enough quality sleep is essential for overall health and sexual vitality. Adequate sleep supports hormone balance and overall well-being.

5. Alcohol and Substance Use

- Excessive alcohol and substance use can negatively affect sexual function. Moderation or abstinence may be necessary for individuals with ED.

6. Smoking Cessation

- Smoking is associated with reduced blood flow and can contribute to ED. Quitting smoking can have a positive impact on sexual health.

7. Stress Reduction

Stress is a common contributor to sexual dysfunction. Managing stress through relaxation techniques, time management, and seeking support when needed can have a positive impact on your sexual well-being.

Remember that small changes in your lifestyle and dietary choices can lead to significant improvements in your overall health and sexual wellness. In the chapters that follow, we'll continue to explore natural approaches to addressing ED, including herbal remedies and the importance of open communication with your partner.

NATURAL APPROACHES TO ERECTILE DYSFUNCTION

Natural approaches to addressing erectile dysfunction (ED) focus on non-medical and non-herbal strategies. These approaches include alternative therapies and lifestyle changes that aim to improve sexual function without the use of prescription medications or herbal remedies. In this chapter, we'll explore some of these natural approaches.

1. Acupuncture

Acupuncture is a traditional Chinese medicine practice that involves inserting thin needles into specific points on the body. Some people find that acupuncture can help improve blood flow and alleviate stress, both of which can have a positive impact on ED.

2. Yoga and Relaxation Techniques

Stress and anxiety are common contributors to ED. Yoga, mindfulness, and relaxation techniques can help reduce stress and promote mental well-being. These practices also improve blood flow and flexibility, which can enhance sexual function.

3. Ayurveda and Traditional Medicine

Ayurveda, the traditional medicine of India, offers a holistic approach to health and wellness. Ayurvedic treatments may include dietary changes, herbs, and lifestyle practices tailored to an individual's constitution, or dosha. Ayurvedic practitioners may recommend specific treatments to address sexual health concerns.

4. Traditional Chinese Medicine (TCM)

Traditional Chinese Medicine employs acupuncture, herbal remedies, and dietary recommendations to address health concerns, including ED. TCM practitioners assess an individual's overall health and aim to balance the body's energy, or Qi, to promote well-being.

5. Homeopathy

Homeopathy is a system of alternative medicine that uses highly diluted substances to stimulate the body's natural healing processes. Some homeopathic remedies are believed to support sexual health and address ED. Consult with a qualified homeopath for personalized recommendations.

These natural approaches are intended to complement other strategies and treatments for ED. It's important to remember that what works for one person may not work for another, and results may vary. Consult with a healthcare professional or alternative medicine practitioner to explore these natural approaches to ED and determine which may be most suitable for your individual needs.

In the following chapters, we will discuss how to combine medical, herbal, and natural approaches to address ED and provide guidance on communicating with your partner as you navigate this journey together.

COMBINING MEDICAL AND HERBAL APPROACHES

Erectile dysfunction (ED) can have multiple underlying causes, both physical and psychological. The holistic approach to addressing ED often involves a combination of medical, herbal, and natural interventions. In this chapter, we'll explore how these different approaches can be combined to create a comprehensive strategy for managing ED.

1. Integrative Strategies

Integrative medicine combines conventional medical treatments with complementary and alternative therapies, such as herbal remedies. By working with a healthcare professional who specializes in integrative medicine, you can create a tailored treatment plan that incorporates the best of both worlds.

2. The Role of Healthcare Professionals

Consulting with healthcare professionals who specialize in sexual health is crucial. They can help you navigate the complexities of combining medical and herbal treatments, ensuring that they are safe and effective for your individual needs.

3. Herbal Supplements and Conventional Treatments

In some cases, herbal supplements can complement prescription medications. For example, a healthcare professional may recommend a specific herbal remedy alongside a prescription medication to enhance the effects. However, it's essential to communicate openly with your healthcare provider about all treatments you're using to avoid potential interactions.

4. Lifestyle and Dietary Recommendations

Combining medical and herbal approaches with lifestyle and dietary changes can have a synergistic effect on ED. For example, improving your diet, engaging in regular physical activity, and practicing stress reduction techniques can enhance the effectiveness of both medical and herbal interventions.

5. Case Studies of Successful Integration

Real-life case studies illustrate how individuals have successfully combined medical and herbal approaches to overcome ED. These stories serve as examples of what's possible and can offer insights into how different strategies can be tailored to individual needs.

By taking an integrative approach to managing ED, you can benefit from the strengths of both conventional and natural treatments. However, it's essential to work closely with a qualified healthcare professional who can provide guidance and ensure that the combination of treatments is safe and suitable for you.

In the following chapters, we will explore the importance of open communication with your partner and healthcare provider as you embark on this journey, and provide resources for continued support and information.

COMMUNICATING WITH YOUR PARTNER

Erectile dysfunction (ED) doesn't just affect the individual experiencing it; it can also have an impact on their partner and the overall dynamics of the relationship. Open and empathetic communication is key to addressing ED together. In this chapter, we'll explore the importance of discussing ED with your partner, providing emotional support, and fostering understanding.

1. The Importance of Open Communication

Discussing ED with your partner can be challenging, but it's a crucial step. By opening up about your experiences and feelings, you can alleviate anxiety and stress, as well as foster intimacy and emotional connection.

2. Setting the Right Environment

Choosing the right time and place for the conversation is important. Create a relaxed and supportive environment where both you and your partner can express your thoughts and feelings without judgment.

3. Exploring Emotional Impact

ED can affect self-esteem and confidence. Both you and your partner should acknowledge the emotional impact of ED and be empathetic to each other's feelings.

4. Reassuring Your Partner

Your partner may be feeling a range of emotions, including worry, frustration, or self-blame. Reassure them that ED is a common issue and is not a reflection of their desirability or your love for them.

5. Discussing Treatment Options

If you're considering treatment options, involve your partner in the decision-making process. Discuss potential treatments and their impact on your relationship. Having your partner's input can make the journey more manageable.

6. Exploring Intimacy Beyond Sexual Activity

Sexual intimacy is just one aspect of a relationship. Explore other ways to maintain intimacy, such as cuddling, spending quality time together, and engaging in activities that bring you closer emotionally.

7. Seeking Professional Help as a Couple

If ED is causing significant strain in your relationship, it may be beneficial to seek professional help as a couple. Couples' therapy or counseling can provide a safe space for both of you to express your concerns and work through relationship challenges.

8. Building a Strong Support System

Lean on your partner for support, and encourage them to do the same. Together, you can build a strong support system that helps you navigate the challenges of ED.

9. Celebrating Small Wins

Acknowledge and celebrate any progress or improvements along the way. These small wins can boost your confidence and strengthen your bond.

Effective communication with your partner is essential as you address ED together. By discussing your experiences, emotions, and treatment options openly, you can reduce the emotional impact of ED and create a supportive and empathetic environment in your relationship.

In the following chapters, we will provide resources for continued support and information as you navigate this journey, whether you choose medical, herbal, or natural approaches to address ED.

EMPOWERMENT AND LONG-TERM WELLNESS

Your journey to addressing erectile dysfunction (ED) is not just about finding a solution; it's also about taking control of your sexual health and overall well-being for the long term. In this chapter, we'll explore how you can empower yourself, set realistic goals, and celebrate successes as you work towards sustained wellness.

1. Taking Charge of Your Sexual Health

Empowerment begins with taking control of your sexual health. This includes making informed decisions, seeking professional help, and being an active participant in your treatment plan.

2. Continual Self-assessment and Monitoring

Stay attuned to your body and emotional well-being. Periodically assess the progress of your treatment and make adjustments as needed. Regular self-assessment can help you identify changes and improvements.

3. Setting Realistic Goals and Expectations

Recovery from ED may be a journey with ups and downs. Setting realistic goals and expectations can help you stay motivated and prevent unnecessary disappointment.

4. Celebrating Successes and Progress

Even small achievements in your journey to addressing ED are worth celebrating. Recognize your progress, whether it's an improved sexual experience, reduced anxiety, or a more robust connection with your partner.

5. Resources for Ongoing Support and Information

Continued support is crucial for long-term wellness. Seek resources, whether it's from healthcare professionals, support groups, or educational materials, to stay informed and connected.

6. Resilience and Adaptation

ED is a common issue, and it can be managed successfully. Building resilience and adaptability can help you face challenges and changes that may arise in your journey to long-term wellness.

7. Emotional Intelligence and Self-awareness

Developing emotional intelligence and self-awareness can contribute to healthier relationships and improved emotional well-being. These skills can be particularly helpful as you navigate the emotional impact of ED.

8. Maintaining Healthy Lifestyle Choices

Continue to make healthy lifestyle choices that support your overall well-being. This includes maintaining a balanced diet, engaging in regular physical activity, and managing stress.

9. Seeking Professional Guidance

As you continue your journey, don't hesitate to consult with healthcare professionals, therapists, or counselors when needed. They can offer guidance and support to help you maintain long-term wellness.

Addressing ED is not just about finding a short-term solution; it's about creating a sustainable path to wellness. Empower yourself with knowledge, self-awareness, and resilience as you work toward achieving your long-term wellness goals.

In the conclusion of this book, we will summarize the key takeaways and provide a final message of encouragement for your journey towards a healthier, more fulfilling sexual life.

CONCLUSION

In the journey to address erectile dysfunction (ED), you've embarked on a path of self-discovery, empowerment, and improved sexual wellness. This comprehensive guide, "Healing Intimacy," has provided you with a wealth of information on medical, herbal, and natural approaches to managing ED, as well as the importance of open communication with your partner and healthcare provider.

Addressing ED is not just about finding a solution; it's about taking control of your sexual health and overall well-being. By combining medical treatments, herbal remedies, and holistic approaches, you have the tools to navigate the challenges of ED and find a path to sustained wellness.

Throughout this book, you've learned about the importance of open communication with your partner, setting realistic goals, and celebrating successes. You've discovered the significance of self-assessment, resilience, and adaptability as you work towards long-term wellness.

Remember that you are not alone in this journey. ED is a common issue, and with the right knowledge, determination, and support, you can regain your sexual vitality and strengthen the bonds of intimacy that make life rich and fulfilling.

As you continue your path to long-term wellness, seek professional guidance when needed, maintain healthy lifestyle choices, and stay connected to resources and support that can provide ongoing information and assistance.

Your journey to address ED is a testament to your commitment to a healthier, more fulfilling sexual life. Keep moving forward with confidence and resilience, and may the path to healing intimacy bring you the joy and satisfaction you deserve.

ABOUT THE AUTHOR

Alex Usifo

Dr. Alex Usifo is a highly respected researcher with over two decades of experience in the field of medicine. I have made significant contributions to the medical field through her clinical work, research, and her role in mentoring the next generation of medical professionals. I have published numerous articles in reputable medical journals and has been at the forefront of groundbreaking research in areas such as cardiovascular medicine and preventive healthcare.

My motivation as an author of medical books is to bridge the gap between medical knowledge and patient understanding. She is deeply committed to making complex medical concepts accessible to the general public and to healthcare professionals seeking to expand their knowledge.

This book covers a wide range of medical topics, from comprehensive guides on specific medical conditions and their treatments to books focusing on wellness, nutrition, and lifestyle choices for maintaining optimal health. My works provide valuable insights for patients, caregivers, and healthcare practitioners alike.

As a medical author, my work serves as a valuable resource for those seeking to better understand medical conditions, treatment options, and the importance of maintaining good health. Her dedication to improving healthcare literacy and her contributions to medical literature have positively impacted countless lives.

www.ingramcontent.com/pod-product-compliance
Lightning Source LLC
Chambersburg PA
CBHW071048260726
48661CB00007B/3198